Build a

Kitchen

Prevent Sickness with Nature's Medicine Cabinet

By: Keith Holmes

The First Vegan World Boxing Champion

Two Time World Champion

Health & Wellness Mentor

Fitness Expert

Introduction

My name is Keith Holmes, and my journey to optimal health began over 30 years ago when I made a life-changing decision—to adopt a vegan lifestyle. At the time, I was a professional boxer competing at the highest level, and many doubted whether I could maintain my strength, endurance, and performance without consuming meat, dairy, or processed supplements. Not only did I prove them wrong, but I became stronger, healthier, and more resilient than ever.

I went on to become a two-time world boxing champion, a two-time United States boxing champion, and a Maryland State champion. More importantly, I became the first vegan world boxing champion in history. My success in the ring was not just about skill and discipline—it was about what I put into my body. By fueling myself with natural, plant-based foods and healing herbs, I never lacked nutrients like protein and iron. Over time, I realized that my diet didn't just enhance my athletic performance—it also protected me from sickness, inflammation, and chronic disease.

For the last 20 years, I have not been sick—not even with a common cold. While many in my family have battled diabetes, high blood pressure, obesity, and cancer, I have remained in peak health, free from these illnesses. This book is a reflection of my journey, my research, and the natural healing knowledge I've gathered over the years. It is my way of sharing the blueprint for longevity and disease prevention through food and herbs.

In these pages, you will learn how to build a natural remedy 'hospital' in your own kitchen, using everyday herbs like ginger, turmeric, burdock root, ashwagandha, and more. You will hear testimonials from those I have mentored and discover how simple lifestyle changes can transform your health. My goal is not just to help you avoid illness—but to empower you to take control of your well-being, naturally.

"Build a Hospital in Your Kitchen"

Prevent Sickness with Nature's Medicine Cabinet

Family traditions have shaped countless lives throughout history. Customs and beliefs have often blinded families to the reality of traditional holidays, birthdays, and other gatherings, where one thing remains consistent: the same food.

Until I was about twenty-five years old, I couldn't see the problems that often arose within families who upheld these traditions. But once it became clear to me, I took a bold step in a new direction. I walked away from the very thing I knew was making my family—and countless others—sick: the diet. The alcohol, drugs, chicken, turkey, seafood, beef, pork, cheese, milk, eggs, white sugar, and white bread were all contributing to poor health.

When I heard doctors say, "It's hereditary. It runs in the family," it hit me like a ton of bricks. The sickness ran in the family because the family shared the same diet and lifestyle. It all made sense, and that realization sparked a change in my mind and my lifestyle.

I knew I had to do something different—not just for myself but for everyone I could reach. I wanted to create a new kind of tradition—a tradition of health and wellness rooted in nature. That's when I set out to build a natural remedy hospital right in my own kitchen. Instead of waiting to get sick and looking for cures, I focused on prevention by incorporating natural herbs and ingredients like ginger, turmeric, burdock root, and ashwagandha root into my daily routine.

This eBook will teach you how to do the same—how to stock your kitchen with powerful, natural remedies that help your body stay strong and resilient. It's not just about curing sickness—it's about building a lifestyle that keeps sickness at bay.

For generations, my family—like many others—followed traditions that shaped not only our culture but also our health. Our tables were always filled with the same foods: meat, milk, eggs, cheese, white bread, and plenty of sugary treats. Drinking alcohol was a common practice, and big, hearty meals were a way of life. But behind the smiles and laughter, sickness was quietly taking root.

My family was stricken with diabetes, high blood pressure, obesity, and even cancer. These diseases didn't just appear out of nowhere—they were the result of lifestyle choices passed down through generations. I used to hear doctors say that these conditions were "hereditary," but I eventually realized that what was truly hereditary wasn't just genetics—it was our eating habits and lifestyle choices.

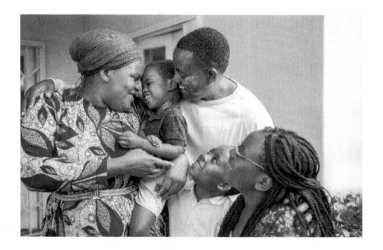

The Philosophy of Prevention:

Building Health from the Inside Out

As a fighter, I took pride in my physical condition, but I wasn't immune to the effects of my diet. During training, I used to catch colds frequently, fighting off illness while preparing for fights. At first, I didn't connect the dots between my diet and my frequent bouts of sickness. It wasn't until I made a conscious decision to walk away from the very foods that had been ingrained in me since childhood that I saw a radical change. The colds stopped. My energy levels increased. I didn't just feel better—I became healthier from the inside out.

I don't have high blood pressure, diabetes, or cancer. I attribute that not just to luck or genetics but to making the conscious choice to break free from harmful traditions. By eliminating meat, dairy and processed foods from my life, I took control of my health. Instead of accepting illness as an inevitable part of aging or family history, I embraced prevention as a way of life.

Diabetes is $110 billion dollar industry

If you were to ask me to wright you a diet that will give you diabetes, I would send you to the American diabetic association website and you can download their guild lines and follow that and you will be on your way to becoming a diabetic

They recommend that you eat oatmeal , a glass of orange juice with natural honey and crushed brown sugar which has all glycemic carbohydrates . That will make your blood sugar spike then you will need an insulin diet.

It's like stealing your car then selling you a car alarm system

To get rid of diabetes, you have to unclog the ducks of the pancreas. It's clogged with carbonic acid.

Why We Stay Sick

The reality is that many families unknowingly pass down cycles of sickness because they pass down the same eating habits. These traditions are often so ingrained that we don't think to question them. We celebrate holidays and milestones with the same heavy, processed meals and think nothing of it. But those choices take a toll— sometimes slowly, sometimes suddenly.

When we eat foods that clog our arteries, burden our organs, and spike our blood sugar, we are essentially inviting sickness into our bodies. And when everyone around us does the same, it feels normal—even when it's far from healthy. That's why I decided to build a new tradition: one centered on prevention and vibrant health.

Maintaining Good Health:
A Daily Commitment

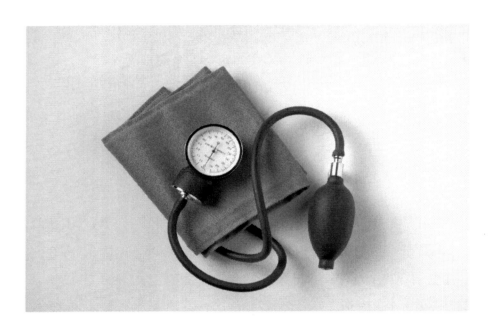

Good health doesn't come from a quick fix or a trendy diet—it's the result of consistent, intentional choices. Every morning, I start my day by drinking natural herbs like turmeric and ginger, which help reduce inflammation throughout my body. During the day, I incorporate other herbs like ashwagandha for prostate health, milk thistle for liver support, burdock root, and sarsaparilla for their rich iron content.

These herbs are not just remedies—they are essential tools for maintaining balance and vitality. By nourishing my body with what it truly needs, I give it the power to fight off disease before it even has a chance to take hold. That's the philosophy of prevention: building a lifestyle that makes sickness unwelcome in the first place.

Breaking the Cycle

The way I see it, we have a choice: to keep passing down habits that make us sick or to start new traditions rooted in wellness. We can build a natural remedy hospital right in our kitchens, using the gifts that nature provides to keep our bodies strong and resilient. I broke the cycle in my family, and now I'm here to help you do the same.

Doctors are able to determine your life span because of your lifestyle.

Personal Story and Inspiration

My journey into veganism started 30 years ago, and it wasn't just a change in diet—it was a transformation of mind, body, and spirit. I didn't know it at the time, but this decision would be the foundation of my lifelong commitment to health and wellness.

Back then, I was searching for something that would give me an edge as a fighter. I wanted to be stronger, faster, and healthier. I'd grown tired of catching colds during training, feeling run down when I needed to be at my peak. I knew something had to change, so I took a bold step away from the foods I'd grown up eating—meat, dairy, processed sugars—and embraced a plant-based lifestyle.

Around that same time, I became more inquisitive about the Bible, especially the scriptures that speak of herbs as food. One verse, in particular, stood out to me: "And God said, Behold, I have given you every herb bearing seed, which is upon the face of all the earth…" That passage resonated with me on a deep level, and I realized that herbs were meant to nourish and heal us. From that point on, I made herbs an essential part of my life.

Herbs have been with me for about 20 years now, and they've proven their worth time and time again. I'll never forget one experience that solidified my commitment to this lifestyle. While training, I suffered an injury to my leg, and my knee became inflamed. The soreness made it hard to move, and I knew I couldn't afford to be sidelined. I'd heard about the anti-inflammatory properties of turmeric, so I mixed it with a pinch of black pepper and drank it regularly. Within a few days, the soreness was gone. That was the turning point for me—I knew this lifestyle wasn't just a temporary change but a permanent commitment.

As I continued my vegan path, I noticed that I wasn't catching colds anymore. My body was stronger, my endurance was better, and my overall well-being had improved drastically. I also started doing regular cleanses and detoxes with homemade green drinks packed with chlorophyll to oxygenate my body. These practices helped me stay rejuvenated and feeling at my best, even through the most demanding training regimens.

Looking back, I realize that stepping away from traditional eating habits wasn't just a physical change—it was a complete mindset shift. I took control of my health by choosing to nourish my body with natural, plant-based foods and powerful herbs. I didn't just accept the idea that sickness was a part of life. I chose to live differently, and that choice has kept me healthy, resilient, and thriving for decades.

Now, I'm on a mission to share what I've learned, to help others break free from cycles of illness and discover the power of building a natural remedy hospital right in their own kitchens. If I can do it, so can you.

Scientific Insights and Expert Opinions:

Harnessing Nature's Power

For centuries, cultures around the world have relied on natural herbs to maintain health and treat ailments. Modern science is finally catching up, providing evidence for what ancient wisdom has long known: nature provides powerful tools for maintaining health. In this section, we'll explore the scientific research behind some of the most effective herbs and break down why they work so well in the body.

Turmeric: The Anti-Inflammatory Powerhouse

One of the most researched and revered herbs is turmeric, a golden-yellow root native to South Asia. Its primary active compound, curcumin, is responsible for its anti-inflammatory and antioxidant properties. Research has shown that curcumin:

• Reduces Inflammation: Curcumin blocks molecules that trigger inflammation, such as nuclear factor-kappa B (NF-κB), which is linked to chronic inflammation and diseases like arthritis and cancer.

• Boosts Antioxidant Capacity: It neutralizes free radicals while boosting the body's own antioxidant enzymes.

• Improves Brain Function: Studies suggest that curcumin may increase brain-derived neurotrophic factor (BDNF), which supports brain health and may reduce the risk of neurodegenerative diseases.

• Supports Heart Health: Curcumin improves the function of the endothelium (the lining of blood vessels), reducing the risk of heart disease.

However, curcumin on its own has low bioavailability, meaning it isn't easily absorbed by the body. That's why it's often combined with black pepper, which contains piperine. Piperine can increase curcumin absorption by up to 2,000%,

Expert Opinion:

Dr. Michael Greger, a renowned nutrition expert and author of How Not to Die, emphasizes the importance of consuming turmeric with black pepper to maximize its health benefits. He explains that the combination not only fights inflammation but also protects cells from oxidative stress.

Ginger: Nature's Digestive and Anti-Inflammatory Aid

Ginger, another powerful root, has been used for thousands of years to treat nausea, digestive issues, and inflammation. The bioactive compound gingerol is largely responsible for its medicinal effects. Scientific studies reveal that ginger:

• **Reduces Muscle Pain and Soreness**: Regular consumption can reduce exercise-induced muscle pain.

• **Fights Infections**: Gingerol has strong antibacterial and antiviral properties, making it effective against respiratory infections.

• Supports Digestive Health: Ginger speeds up gastric emptying, reducing discomfort from indigestion.

• **Lowers Blood Sugar Levels**: A 2015 study published in the Journal of Complementary and Integrative Medicine found that ginger significantly reduced fasting blood sugar levels in people with type 2 diabetes.

How to Prepare and Take Herbs for Maximum Benefits

When using herbs as natural medicine, the preparation method is just as important as the herbs themselves. Proper preparation allows the body to absorb the nutrients and healing compounds effectively. Below is a simple guide to brewing herbal teas for optimal health.

Basic Herbal Tea Preparation

1. Measure the Herbs: Use one teaspoon of dried herbs per eight-ounce cup of water. If using fresh herbs, double the amount.

2. Boil the Water: Bring the water to a boil in a pot or kettle.

3. Steep the Herbs: Turn off the burner and add the herbs to the hot water. Let them sit for five minutes to extract the medicinal properties.

4. Strain and Drink: Pour the tea through a strainer into a cup and enjoy while warm.

Herbal Blends for Maximum Health

I often mix powerful herb combinations to boost their healing effects. Here are some of my go-to blends:

✅ **Blood Cleanser & Detox Blend:**

• **Pau D'Arco** (supports immunity)

• **Dandelion** (cleanses the liver)

• **Burdock Root** (removes toxins from the blood)

• **Red Clover** (supports the lymphatic system)

✅ **Anti-Inflammatory & Digestive Blend:**

• **Turmeric** (reduces inflammation)

• **A sprinkle of Black Pepper** (enhances turmeric absorption)

• **Ginger** (supports digestion and circulation)

Daily Herbal Routine

Drinking herbal teas regularly can help prevent illness and maintain health. I personally drink my herbal blends throughout the day, focusing on anti-inflammatory teas in the morning and detoxifying blends in the evening.

Consistency is key—your body thrives when given the right tools to heal itself naturally. Start incorporating these herbs into your daily routine and experience the transformation!

Expert Opinion:

Dr. Josh Axe, a certified doctor of natural medicine and clinical nutritionist, advocates for using ginger daily to support digestion and reduce inflammation. He points out that even small amounts can significantly impact overall health and recovery from physical activity.

Ashwagandha: The Adaptogenic Wonder

Ashwagandha is an ancient medicinal herb classified as an adaptogen, meaning it helps the body manage stress. Its active compounds, including withanolides, offer numerous health benefits:

• **Reduces Stress and Anxiety**: Studies show that ashwagandha lowers cortisol levels, the stress hormone, helping to combat chronic stress.

• **Supports Prostate Health**: Its anti-inflammatory properties may protect against prostate enlargement and promote urinary function.

• **Enhances Muscle Strength and Recovery:** Research published in the Journal of the International Society of Sports Nutrition found that supplementing with ashwagandha significantly increased muscle mass and strength.

• **Boosts Immunity**: As an adaptogen, it supports the immune system by reducing the impact of stress on the body.

Expert Opinion:

Dr. Andrew Weil, a pioneer in integrative medicine, highlights ashwagandha's potential to enhance vitality and well-being. He notes that its balancing effects on hormones make it a valuable addition to a wellness routine.

Milk Thistle: The Liver Protector

Milk thistle is well known for its liver-protective properties, thanks to the active compound silymarin. Research shows that silymarin:

• **Supports Liver Detoxification**: It enhances the production of glutathione, a powerful antioxidant that detoxifies harmful substances.

• **Reduces Liver Inflammation**: Studies suggest it may benefit people with liver conditions such as fatty liver disease and hepatitis.

• **Improves Liver Function**: Regular use can help the liver regenerate and repair damaged tissue.

Expert Opinion:

Dr. Tori Hudson, a naturopathic physician, recommends milk thistle for individuals exposed to toxins or dealing with liver stress. She believes that its ability to enhance detoxification pathways makes it essential for maintaining liver health.

Burdock Root: Blood Purifier and Detox Agent

Burdock root has long been used to cleanse the blood and support organ function. Its benefits include:

• **Detoxifying the Blood**: Burdock root helps eliminate toxins through improved circulation and enhanced lymphatic drainage.

• **Supporting Skin Health**: Its anti-inflammatory and antibacterial properties aid in treating skin conditions like eczema and acne.

• **Rich in Antioxidants:** Contains quercetin, luteolin, and phenolic acids that fight oxidative stress.

Expert Opinion:

Dr. Edward Group, a global leader in holistic health, praises burdock root for its blood-cleansing abilities. He advocates incorporating it into detox routines to help maintain a clean internal environment.

Sarsaparilla: Iron-Rich and Anti-Inflammatory

Sarsaparilla has been valued for its high iron content and ability to support blood health. Its benefits include:

• **Boosting Iron Levels**: A valuable herb for individuals prone to anemia or low iron.

• **Anti-Inflammatory Effects:** Contains compounds that reduce swelling and pain, aiding in joint health.

• **Promoting Kidney Health**: Acts as a diuretic to support the elimination of excess fluids and toxins.

Expert Opinion:

Herbalist Rosemary Gladstar, known as the "godmother of modern herbalism," often recommends sarsaparilla for its detoxifying and nourishing properties, especially for those struggling with fatigue or iron deficiency.

Pau D'Arco (Tabebuia impetiginosa) – Pau D'Arco is derived from the inner bark of a South American tree and has been traditionally used for its antimicrobial, antifungal, and immune-boosting properties.

• **Anti-Fungal & Anti-Bacterial:** Studies show Pau D'Arco contains lapachol and beta-lapachone, compounds that help fight Candida overgrowth, bacterial infections, and parasites.

• **Immune System Support**: It stimulates the production of white blood cells, strengthening immune defenses.

• **Anti-Inflammatory**: Helps reduce chronic inflammation, making it beneficial for arthritis, joint pain, and inflammatory bowel conditions.

• **Cancer-Fighting Potential**: Some research suggests that Pau D'Arco may have anticancer properties by inhibiting tumor cell growth.

• **Digestive Health**: Used to promote gut health and relieve issues like leaky gut, bloating, and infections.

Expert Opinion:

Dr. Andrew Weil, an integrative medicine specialist, acknowledges Pau D'Arco's antifungal properties and its traditional use for immune support. However, he advises using it in moderation, as high doses may cause nausea or interfere with blood clotting.

Dandelion (Taraxacum officinale) –
Dandelion is a powerful herb commonly used for liver detoxification, digestive health, and reducing water retention.

• **Liver Detoxifier**: Dandelion root supports liver function by increasing bile production and flushing out toxins.

• **Diuretic & Kidney Support**: Helps eliminate excess water and sodium without depleting potassium levels.

• **Rich in Antioxidants**: Contains polyphenols and beta-carotene, which help protect cells from oxidative stress.

• **Supports Digestion**: Acts as a prebiotic, promoting gut health and feeding beneficial bacteria.

• **Blood Sugar Regulation**: Some studies suggest dandelion may help regulate blood sugar and support insulin sensitivity.

10 amazing health benefits of
PUMPKIN SEEDS

1. the only seed that is alkaline-forming
2. can reduce levels of LDL cholesterol
3. 100 g seeds provide 30 g protein
4. used traditionally to kill parasites!
5. reduce inflammation for arthritis
6. prevent kidney stone formation
7. good for prostate health
8. promote good sleep
9. filled with minerals
10. high in zinc.

Herbs for Detoxing & Removing Parasites

The following herbs work synergistically to help cleanse the body of toxins, eliminate parasites, and support overall gut health. They can be used together by steeping one teaspoon of each herb in 8 oz of boiling water for 10-15 minutes.

1. Wormwood (Artemisia absinthium)

• **Powerful Antiparasitic**: Wormwood is one of the most effective herbs for eliminating intestinal worms, including tapeworms and roundworms.

• **Liver & Digestive Support**: Stimulates bile production and aids digestion.

• **Anti-Microbial**: Helps fight infections, including bacterial and fungal overgrowth.

> **Usage:** Drink as a tea or take in capsule form. Avoid prolonged use, as it can be toxic in high doses.

2. Senna Leaves (Senna alexandrina)

- **Strong Laxative**: Helps flush out waste and parasites by promoting bowel movements.

- **Colon Cleanser**: Works well for short-term detox programs.

Usage: Best used occasionally to avoid dependency. Combine with hydrating herbs to prevent dehydration.

3. **Black Walnut (Juglans nigra)**

• **Kills Parasites**: Contains juglone, a compound known to eliminate parasites, especially intestinal worms.

• **Supports Gut Health:** Helps repair intestinal lining and fights Candida.

• **Anti-Fungal & Anti-Bacterial:** Useful for bacterial infections and fungal overgrowth.

Usage: Used as a tincture or tea. Avoid excessive use due to its potency.

4. **Cloves** (Syzygium aromaticum)

• **Destroys Parasite Eggs**: One of the few herbs that can kill parasite larvae and eggs, preventing reinfestation.

• **Antiseptic & Anti-Inflammatory**: Helps soothe digestive discomfort and bloating.

• **Boosts Circulation**: Supports overall body detoxification.

Usage: Can be brewed into tea or taken as a powdered supplement. Best when combined with other antiparasitic herbs.

How to Use These Herbs Together for Detoxing & Parasite Removal

Parasite Cleanse Tea Recipe:

1. Boil 8 oz of water.

2. Add one teaspoon each of wormwood, senna leaves, black walnut hull, and cloves.

3. Let steep for 10-15 minutes before straining.

4. Drink once daily in the early morning on an empty stomach 2-3 days per week (take a break after two weeks).

Additional Tips:

• **For best results, follow a clean diet (avoid sugar and processed foods, which feed parasites).**

• **Pair with probiotics to restore gut balance.**

• Consult a healthcare professional if you have any medical conditions or are pregnant/nursing.

This blend helps cleanse the intestines, kill parasites, and support the body's natural detoxification process.

Foods and Drinks to Avoid While Detoxing with These Herbs

When detoxing with Wormwood, Senna Leaves, Black Walnut, Cloves, Pau D'Arco, and Dandelion, it's important to avoid foods and drinks that can hinder the cleansing process or feed parasites.

1. No Alcohol or Drugs

Alcohol strains the liver and weakens detoxification. It also feeds harmful bacteria and yeast (like Candida).

Recreational drugs and pharmaceuticals (unless prescribed and necessary) should be minimized because they place extra stress on the liver and kidneys.

2. No Processed Sugars or Refined Carbohydrates

• Parasites thrive on sugar—cutting it out helps starve them.

- **Avoid:**

- White sugar, high-fructose corn syrup, artificial sweeteners

- White bread, pastries, cakes, cookies

- Sweetened drinks (soda, energy drinks, store-bought fruit juices)

3. No Dairy Products

- Dairy can be mucus-forming, which makes it harder for the body to eliminate toxins.

- Milk, cheese, yogurt, and butter may also contain hormones and antibiotics that interfere with detoxing.

4. No Fried or Greasy Foods

- These foods slow digestion and burden the liver.

- **Avoid**:

- Fast food

• Deep-fried foods (French fries, fried chicken, potato chips)

• Processed oils (vegetable, canola, soybean)

5. No Meat or Animal Products

• Meat, especially red meat and pork, is hard to digest and can create an acidic environment where parasites thrive.

• **Avoid**:

• Beef, pork, chicken

• Processed meats (hot dogs, bacon, sausage)

6. No Caffeinated Beverages

• Coffee and energy drinks can dehydrate the body and put stress on the adrenal glands.

• If you need a warm drink, opt for herbal teas instead.

7. No Tap Water or Sugary Drinks

• Tap water may contain chlorine, fluoride, and heavy metals that can disrupt detoxification.

• Instead, drink spring water, distilled water, or herbal teas.

What to Eat Instead?

• **Hydrating foods**: Fresh fruits (berries, apples, citrus)

• **Alkalizing vegetables**: Leafy greens (kale, spinach, arugula), cucumbers, zucchini

• **Healthy fats**: Avocados, coconut oil, flaxseeds, walnuts

• **Herbal teas**: Ginger, turmeric, peppermint, dandelion, Pau D'Arco

One of the biggest contributors to illness is excess mucus and chronic inflammation in the body. These two factors are at the root of many diseases, including high blood pressure, diabetes, arthritis, and even cancer. The good news is that by eliminating the sources of excess mucus and inflammation, the body can heal naturally.

What Causes Excess Mucus?

• **Dairy Products** – Milk, cheese, and yogurt cause mucus buildup, leading to congestion.

• **Processed Foods** – Refined sugars and artificial additives trigger inflammation and excess mucus.

• **Meat and Fried Foods** – These foods slow down digestion and contribute to mucus production.

• **Environmental Toxins** – Pollutants, smoke, and chemicals irritate the body and increase mucus.

When mucus builds up, it blocks proper oxygen flow in the body and prevents the organs from functioning properly. This can lead to:

• **Respiratory Issues** – Asthma, bronchitis, sinus infections, and chronic cough.

• **Digestive Problems** – Constipation, bloating, and acid reflux.

• **Joint Pain** – Excess mucus contributes to inflammation in the joints.

Inflammation: The Root of Most Sickness

Inflammation is the body's natural defense mechanism. When you get a cut, the area swells up as part of the healing process. But chronic inflammation, caused by poor diet and lifestyle, leads to disease.

Common Diseases Linked to Chronic Inflammation:

• **High Blood Pressure** – Inflammation damages blood vessels, leading to hypertension.

• **Diabetes** – Chronic inflammation disrupts insulin function.

• **Arthritis** – Inflammation in the joints leads to pain and stiffness.

• **Cancer** – Long-term inflammation can damage cells and lead to tumor growth.

How to Remove Mucus and Reduce Inflammation

The key to healing the body is to eliminate mucus-forming foods and adopt an anti-inflammatory diet.

Powerful Anti-Mucus and Anti-Inflammatory Foods:

• **Turmeric** – Contains curcumin, which reduces inflammation and improves blood circulation.

• **Ginger** – A natural decongestant that breaks down mucus in the lungs and digestive tract.

• **Sea Moss** – Removes mucus from the body and provides 92 essential minerals.

• **Burdock Root** – Purifies the blood and helps clear mucus buildup.

• **Sarsaparilla** – High in iron and excellent for cleansing the body.

• **Leafy Greens** – High in chlorophyll, which detoxifies and reduces inflammation.

The Benefits of Removing Mucus and Inflammation

When you remove mucus and reduce inflammation, you will experience:

✅ **Better breathing** – No more chronic congestion or sinus problems.

✅ **Increased energy** – Less inflammation means better blood flow and oxygen to the organs.

✅ **Pain relief** – Reduced inflammation means less joint and muscle pain.

✅ **Improved digestion** – No more bloating, acid reflux, or constipation.

✅ **Faster healing** – With better blood circulation, the body can repair itself naturally.

Final Thought: Let Your Body Heal Itself

Most sickness is not hereditary—it is habitual. When we stop feeding the body harmful foods and give it what it truly needs, the body can heal on its own. Removing mucus and inflammation is one of the most powerful steps toward better health.

Are you ready to cleanse your body and start feeling better? It all starts in your kitchen hospital!

Sea moss contains 92 of the 102 essential minerals the human body needs. These include:

- **Iodine** – Supports thyroid function and hormone regulation.

- **Iron** – Boosts energy and supports oxygen transport in the blood.

- **Magnesium** – Reduces inflammation and supports muscle and nerve function.

- **Calcium** – Strengthens bones and teeth.

- **Zinc** – Boosts immune function and aids wound healing.

- **Potassium** – Regulates blood pressure and supports heart health.

Health Benefits of Sea Moss

1. Boosts Immunity and Fights Inflammation

Sea moss is rich in antioxidants and anti-inflammatory compounds that help the body fight off infections and illnesses.

Scientific Evidence:

• A 2018 study published in Marine Drugs found that sea moss contains bioactive compounds that boost immune function and reduce inflammation.

2. Supports Thyroid Health

The thyroid gland relies on iodine to produce hormones that regulate metabolism, energy levels, and brain function. Sea moss is naturally high in iodine, making it an excellent choice for supporting thyroid health.

Scientific Evidence:

• Research published in the Journal of Medicinal Food in 2014 highlights the importance of seaweed-derived iodine in preventing hypothyroidism.

3. **Improves Digestion and Gut Health**

Sea moss contains prebiotic fiber, which nourishes healthy gut bacteria and aids digestion. It also has mucilage, a gel-like substance that soothes the digestive tract.

Scientific Evidence:

• A 2020 study in BMC Complementary Medicine and Therapies found that sea moss improved gut microbiome diversity and helped reduce inflammation in the intestines.

4. Enhances Skin Health

Sea moss is loaded with collagen-boosting nutrients that help keep skin firm, hydrated, and youthful. It also has antibacterial properties that can help treat acne and skin infections.

Scientific Evidence:

• A 2015 study in Phytotherapy Research found that the sulfated polysaccharides in sea moss have skin-healing and anti-aging properties.

5. Supports Heart Health

The potassium and omega-3 fatty acids in sea moss help regulate blood pressure and lower cholesterol, reducing the risk of heart disease.

Scientific Evidence:

• A 2019 study in the Journal of Applied Phycology showed that sea moss consumption helped lower LDL ("bad") cholesterol and improved overall heart health.

6. Increases Energy and Fights Fatigue

Because sea moss is rich in iron and B vitamins, it helps prevent anemia and boosts energy levels naturally.

Scientific Evidence:

• A 2017 study published in Nutrients found that seaweed-derived iron is highly bioavailable and effective in reducing fatigue.

7. Aids in Weight Loss

The natural fiber in sea moss promotes a feeling of fullness, helping to reduce overeating. It also helps balance metabolism and detoxify the body.

Scientific Evidence:

• A study in Nutrients (2020) found that alginate, a compound in sea moss, reduces fat absorption and promotes weight loss.

How to Use Sea Moss

- Sea Moss Gel: Blend soaked sea moss with water to create a gel. Add it to smoothies, soups, or tea.

- Capsules/Powder: Take sea moss as a supplement for easy consumption.

- Topical Use: Apply sea moss gel to the skin as a natural moisturizer and healing agent.

☐

Final Thoughts

Sea moss is a powerhouse of nutrients with scientifically proven health benefits. By incorporating it into your diet, you can boost immunity, improve digestion, support thyroid health, and promote overall well-being.

Nature has provided everything we need to thrive, and sea moss is one of the best natural tools for maintaining health.

Nature's Blueprint for Health

These herbs are more than just remedies—
they
are nature's blueprint for maintaining health
and vitality. Unlike synthetic drugs that often
come with side effects, these natural
ingredients work in harmony with the body's
systems, providing long-lasting support.

The beauty of natural herbs lies not only in
their power but in their simplicity. They don't
just mask symptoms; they address the root
causes of health issues. By incorporating
them into your daily routine, you build a
foundation of wellness that strengthens the
body from the inside out.

In a world where chronic illness has become
the norm, these natural remedies offer a
pathway to a healthier, more resilient life.
They remind us that health isn't just about
avoiding sickness—it's about embracing a

lifestyle that keeps the body strong, balanced, and thriving.

Final Thoughts and Motivation

When I walk into my kitchen, the first thing I see is my countertop lined with containers of herbs—each one a powerful remedy and a natural defense against sickness. Open my refrigerator, and you'll find fresh herbal drinks, vibrant vegetables, homemade green juices, plant-based milk, and plant-based cheese.

It's not just food; it's medicine.
My kitchen isn't just a place to prepare meals—it's my personal hospital, built on the principles of natural wellness and prevention.

Made in the USA
Middletown, DE
22 April 2025

74500626R00042